The Purpose of this Book.

Many people feel overwhelmed by all the information they hear about CoVid-19. You are worried about getting CoVid and you are worried about what will happen if you become infected or if someone you love becomes infected.

I also understand that for many people, science was never their strength, so this book is written for the general public. As such the real scientists and physicians reading this may think it is too basic for them; however, based upon what I am seeing, I think this book is a good place for many of the scientists and physicians to begin as well.

This book is a brief look at CoVid-19. Where it came from; what tests to get and when; how to reduce your risk of catching CoVid, and more importantly what are the treatments.

Like everything else, thanks to the lawyers, judges and Big Pharma, we begin this book by saying in the American Tradition of CYA; This book is not providing you medical advice and it does not replace your seeing your doctor.

Although, you may want to take this book with you when you see your doctor, since the reason so people are dying with CoVid-19 was first explained by myself in 1994, then 1995, published in a Cardiology Textbook in 1999, more published work in the early 2000's and finally discussed on 20/20 in 2004. Despite all of the presentations and publications patients have continued to be treated as if the only problem was the virus itself.

The reason for so many deaths is the untreated INFLAMMATION and BLOOD CLOTTING occurring in response to the virus, particularly in people who have pre-existing health problems that predispose them to the inflammation and blood clotting killing them.

Our research and more details about SARS-CoV-2 (aka CoVid-19) are discussed in the Unmasking CoViD books written by myself.

Dr. Richard M. Fleming
Physicist – Nuclear Cardiologist
Author of The Inflammation and Cardiovascular
Disease Theory

Table of Contents

Chapter 1 – Viruses are Real – Ignore the Grifters!

One of the many arguments proposed to make people feel better is that viruses aren't real. If they aren't real they can't hurt you and we can automatically return to "normal."

The problem with this approach is that the grifters proposing this argument are making this up on the run. Some of them will tell you that what scientists and physicians have found and are calling viruses is nothing more than the body itself.

These grifters will tell you that the virus is something called an exosome. Exosomes ARE real but they aren't viruses. One of the infamous people promoting this ideal is Dr. Andrew Kaufman. Kaufman like many others claim that the genetic material identified as CoVid-19 is really something made by us. They claim that CoVid-19 is nothing but a hoax designed to control us and take away our personal freedoms.

While I would not argue with the idea that people in power, including many elected officials, are using this opportunity to restrain us and take away personal freedoms, that doesn't mean that the virus isn't real.

"Never let a good crisis go to waste." These words have been spoken by Winston Churchill, Rahm Emanuel, Saul Alinsky, & Machiavelli

In fact, if the elections of 2020 showed us anything, it was that those in power, who proposed not stripping people of their personal freedoms, would be held accountable by those willing to take those freedoms away. The simple use of fear was enough to cost many of these elected officials re-election.

But Kaufman is wrong when he argues that CoVid and other viruses are exosomes. Exosomes are merely packets of material put together by the cells of our body to warn our body of a problem – including viruses like CoVid-19.

Kaufman, like so many others including Robert O Young, who have no training or experience in viruses declare that cells of our body are making these exosomes in response to environmental harm like air and water pollution or 5-G. This argument is faulty on the very surface because it suggests that in response to an external harm, our bodies are making exosomes that cause more harm and killing people. Kaufman's argument is that our body makes harmful exosomes in response to harmful pollution and 5-G. In other words, our bodies are killing us.

Another part of their fallacy arguments is that viruses are made by the red blood cells of our body. This is completely impossible since the red blood cells lack any of the material to make viruses or anything else. Our red blood cells carry our oxygen and help remove carbon dioxide from our body.

Kaufman, Young and others, are willing to sell you their services on line including consultation for a thousand plus dollars an hour.

Yes, Virginia – there may be a Santa Claus – but No, Virginia, Viruses are not exosomes or mutated red blood cells. And No, Dr. Kaufman, CoVid-19 isn't called "19" because there were 18 other corona viruses before this one. It's because it was reported in 2019.

Chapter 2 – This virus has been modified by humans.

There is no doubt that corona viruses are real with the first well-known corona virus being SARS-CoV-1 in 2002.

SARS stands for Severe Acute Respiratory Syndrome, which means that once infected with the virus, the person can experience a severe problem with breathing that occurs suddenly (acute).

This can be the result of either inflammation with fluid accumulating in the airways of the lungs, or blood clots occurring in the lungs interfering with blood flow and our ability to take oxygen from our lungs to our body.

Following the discovery of SARS-CoV-1 (SARS Corona Virus 1) in 2002, a deadlier version infected people in the Middle East in 2012. This particular corona virus, which also produced severe problems with breathing, was called MERS-CoV (Middle East Respiratory Syndrome Corona Virus).

After the initial outbreak of SARS-CoV-1 in 2002 research funded in part by the National Science Foundation (NSF) and the National Institute for Allergy and Infectious (NIAID) Diseases began funding studies looking at the spread of these viruses. The research looked at both how to increase the spread of these viruses as well as limit the spread.

The research showed that the key to limiting the spread of the virus was to shut down international travel and yet, when CoVid-19 hit China late in 2019, this information was not given to the President of the United States - despite taxpayer U.S. money being used to pay for the studies. Nonetheless he shut down international travel.

The paper trail shows involvement by both the U.S. and China Governments as the virus was studied and human modifications were made that increased the ability of the virus to infect people.

The paper trail shows the intentional insertion of an HIV component and a rabies component, both of which appear to have increased the ability of SARS-CoV-2 (CoVid-19) to infect people. These changes are known as "gain-in-function" and if only one change had occurred it could be argued that the change naturally occurred. But for two such changes to have occurred would be astronomical.

In the end this virus does not appear to have been the result of a wet market in China but rather a human-modified virus that escaped from the Wuhan laboratory – either intentionally or by sloppiness.

The result was the same; the release of a human modified virus with increased ability to infect people. Paid for by U.S. taxpayer money.

Chapter 3 – Reducing the spread.

Understanding how a virus moves from person to person is key to finding, stopping and treating the virus.

We all know this is a virus that spreads through the air. It moves from person to person when we cough or sneeze. Most of us have seen the videos of the mucous watery material being expelled when people cough or sneeze and it the size of these watery particles that is critical to understanding the spread.

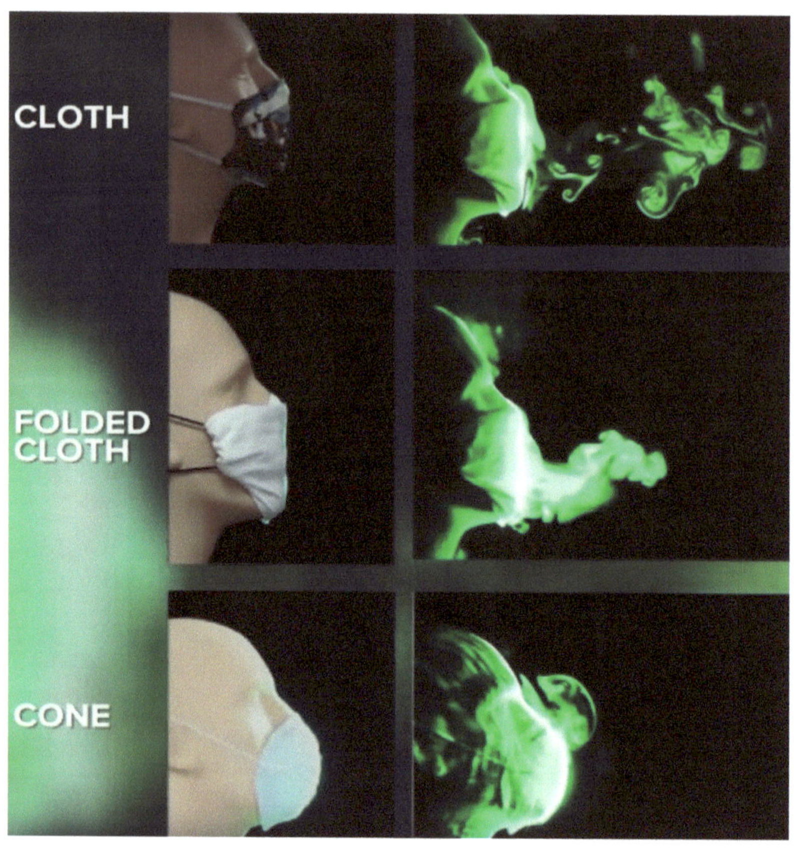

The virus itself needs to be attached to the mucous watery material to successfully pass from person to person. This is the argument for wearing masks.

Yes, wearing a mask reduces the forward movement of the virus with a cough or sneeze but it merely changes the direction of the virus. As a result, remaining in areas where there are a number of people who are contagious can increase the ability of the virus to find you anyway.

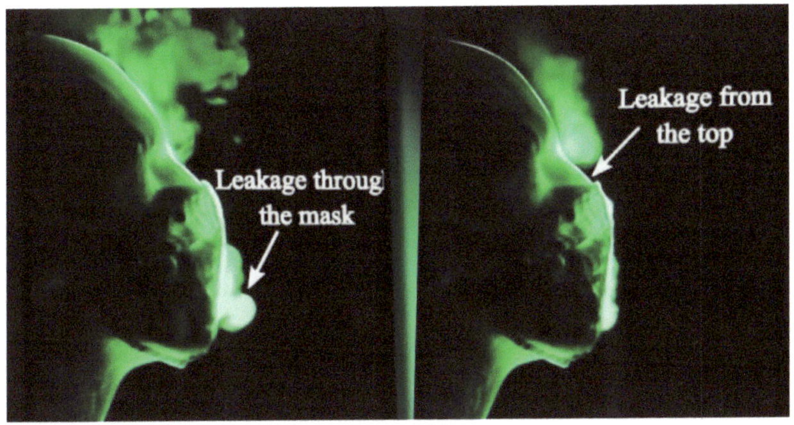

Yes, there is an argument to be made for and against masks. The question is motive. Too many people advocating for masks do so out of fear. Too many people advocating for no masks do so out of fear. The fear is different for the two groups and because they are arguing out of fear – one for fear of dying and the other for fear of losing personal freedoms – there is little true discussion about the benefits or lack of benefit from wearing a mask.

In areas where there are large numbers of people in close proximity that may have been or are coughing or sneezing, there is a greater chance that the virus can be floating about. This is a risk that could be dramatically reduced by following the same practice we do with other viruses. When sick, stay home. Quarantine the sick, not the healthy.

The other and probably the greatest way to reduce the spread of a virus are cleaning our hands and the surfaces where people's hand have been and the surfaces that have been sneezed or coughed upon. However, there is a balance between obsession and cleanliness.

Chapter 4 – Changes in diet and vitamin support.

People with pre-existing conditions that predispose them to dying with CoVid-19 are frequently people who are overweight; have heart disease, diabetes, cancer, high blood pressure, strokes, and other diseases caused by inflammation. The vast majority of these people have the diseases because of diets high in processed and refined foods and/or diets high in saturated fat.

When I first presented the Inflammation and Cardiovascular Disease Theory in 1994, as I mentioned in the Purpose of this Book section, one of the points I made clear was that viruses and bacteria could once again become the number one killer of people by causing inflammation in the blood vessels of the body. That is exactly what CoVid-19 is doing.

The argument about whether people are dying from or with CoVid-19 is moot – i.e. it is unimportant. You cannot die from the inflammation caused by (with) CoVid-19 without getting the infection. The failure of doctors to treat this inflammation and blood clotting explains why the people are dying but it is not the reason the people get (from) CoVid-19.

In most combat sports one of the first things people want to do is learn how to attack. The first thing you are taught is how to defend. You can't attack your opponent if you are lying on the ground. Defense is the first thing to learn. Don't be where the punch or kick is landing. If you're not there, you can't be hurt by it.

The same thing is true for CoVid-19, which means reducing your exposure to it and by having a healthier body so your reaction to it doesn't harm you.

To have a healthier body means knowing what to eat and what to put inside your body and what to keep outside of your body.

The evidence shows that diets that are high in saturated fat and/or high in calories or refined and processed foods have predisposed people to having heart disease, diabetes, cancer, high blood pressure, strokes, or to being overweight. All of these are associated with increased inflammation and blood clots following infection with CoVid-19 leading to death.

One of the major arguments for the reduction in deaths in China and Asian countries has been the use of masks, which may be beneficial. I would argue it is their diet and lifestyle that has resulted in there being less inflammatory disease and fewer deaths.

These same diets are also associated with a better balance of vitamins and minerals known to improve the ability of our bodies to fight off infections. In our research study (NCT04349410) people who ended up in the hospital were given Folate, Magnesium, Calcium Carbonate, Vitamin B6 & B12, DHEA, Vitamin C, Vitamin D3 and Zinc.

Each of these vitamins and minerals have been shown to improve our bodies response to infection and when combined with the other treatments were successful in treating CoVid-19 patients 99.83% of the time.

Chapter 5 – Treatments.

Treating CoVid-19 is not magic; it is science. Unfortunately political and personal differences have made it extremely challenging to find the best treatments for people infected with CoVid-19.

Nothing provides more evidence of this than the arguments surrounding the use of hydroxychloroquine (HCQ) for CoVid. HCQ has been used for decades for malaria but that does not mean that HCQ is only useful for malaria.

No drug is useful for only one purpose. Drugs like minoxidil are used for hair growth but it began and is still used for high blood pressure. Interestingly enough there are some serious side effects associated with minoxidil and close monitoring of the heart is advisable for people on minoxidil. Yet, there has been no effort to stop the use of minoxidil for people who are looking to re-grow hair on their head.

Because no drug, with a couple of very rare exceptions, is used for just one purpose, drugs are usually approved by the FDA for a specific reason and are then used by doctors for a variety of other reasons. That has been the way medicine has always been practiced. If a doctor believes a medication is useful for their patient, and the patient agrees to take the medicine, then the medicine can be used.

Unless you have been living under a rock, you have undoubtedly heard that HCQ may cause problems with the rhythm of your heart and there has been tremendous interference by non-physicians to prevent doctors from using HCQ for CoVid-19 patients.

There is however no evidence to support this concern and blockade of HCQ use. To be clear, HCQ can prolong the QTc interval of the heart. This prolongation could result in life threatening changes in the heart rhythm known as polymorphic ventricular dysrhythmias or torsade de pointes. Despite all the talk, I am aware of no instance where a patient receiving HCQ has had either of these rhythm problems. It is also true that the inflammation associated with CoVid-19 can also prolong the QTc; so the question really becomes is it the use of HCQ or the inflammation caused by the infection that is at fault?

The treatment of SARS-CoV-2 (CoVid-19) is dependent upon where in the cycle of this infection the patient is. Are they in the early phase or a later phase where the inflammation and blood clotting is occurring.

On the next page is my recommended treatment protocol for SARS-CoV-2 focusing on where the patient is in the cycle of infection.

Fleming SARS-CoV-2 Treatment Protocol.

Pre-hospitalization	Hospitalization and Evaluation of SARS-CoV-2 severity on Day 1.	Rx Acute Innate T-cell Cytoxic Immune Response Beginning on Day 1.

→

Symptomatic or High-risk groups.	FMTVDM measurement of SARS-CoV-2.	Initiate Additional Treatment
Begin HCQ, AZT or alternative (Primaquine & Clindamycin) to inhibit viral attachment and replication.	Begin pre-hospitalization Rxs if not already started.	Bronchodilator Rx with β-2 agonist.
Begin Immune supportive Rx including Zn.	ECG and Rx any prolongation of QTc with Esmolol, K, Ca, & Mg.	Consider adding Primaquine 200 mg one time dose if not already given.
Consider combination administration of interferon α-2β treatment with other agents - eg. Atrovent inhalers/ nebulizer; aminoquinoline; clindamycin.	Measure inflammatory & thrombotic markers and treat accordingly to address and prevent clotting and further uncontrolled inflammation.	Immediately add one of the three following treatment regimens to address InflammoThrombotic Response (ITR).
	Do NOT merely leave patient in bed (chair, ambulate, etc.).	(1) Tocilizumab & Interferon α-2β; (2) Primaquine, Clindamycin, Tocilizumab & Interferon α-2β, or (3) Methylprednisolone.

Oxygenation Begin on Day 1.

Evaluate Treatment Response with FMTVDM on Day 3 after 72-hours of Rx.

Delayed Adaptive Humoral Immune & ITR Treatment. Day 3 immediately after FMTVDM.

Use incentive spirometry for Rx and measure of respiratory strength.

With any compromise in ventilatory status begin PRONE positioning of patient.

Consider supplemental oxygen and BiPAP.

Prepare for V-V or V-A ECMO support.

If other measures fail consider ventilatory support with VT not to exceed 5 cc/kg IDBW.

Extubate ASAP!

FMTVDM measurement to determine Rx effect.

(1) Improved. Cont Rx.
(2) Stable. Add next level of Rx.
(3) Deterioration. Change Rx.

Adjust Rx given FMTVDM results.

If further Rx is to be added, select from (1) Tocilizumab & Interferon α-2β; (2) Primaquine, Clindamycin, Tocilizumab & Interferon α-2β, or (3) Methylprednisolone.

Continue to aggressively address inflammatory and clotting disorders including efforts to get patient out of bed (chair, ambulate, etc.) to avoid further thromobotic and inflammatory problems.

Consider passive immunity with plasma with attention directed to potential associated clotting potential.

It is entirely up to you and your doctor on whether these treatments are used. Since these drugs are already FDA approved, in keeping with the practice of medicine, they do not require additional FDA approval. The question is whether political and personal differences will interfere in the practice of medicine and the care of millions around the world.